WWW.OWNERS-GUIDE.COM

# Depression:
# the Mechanical Cause

## How to Rewire Your Brain

### Dr John Bergman

This book is dedicated to those people who have changed their perception of what health is and what disease is. If you change your perception, you change your world. If your perception is that you have a "disease or condition," you will treat that "disease or condition." If you change your perception about "disease" to disease being an intelligent response of your body adapting to toxicity or deficiency, you will then appreciate your body's response and recover health by correcting the deficiencies and eliminating the toxicities.

**How to Create a Health Revolution:**

Depression/Bipolar Disorder

Mechanical Cause and Cure

# *Preface*

It takes a tremendous amount of courage to take charge of your own health. Today in 2014 there is a medical cartel in place that has tremendous political power. This cartel has been established by the Pharmaceutical industry, the largest and most powerful industry on our planet. It is designed to profit from the treatment of disease by using patentable chemicals. It is *not* designed for the optimal health of our population. This book will lay out a step-by-step revolution for the people of our planet to take back our natural state, which is a full, disease-free life. Imagine waking up in the morning in a positive mental state, full of energy, and with the ability to handle stress in a healthy manner. Of course every human being will experience stressors, either physical, chemical or emotional stress; normal emotional and physical reactions to stress are now being labeled as *medical conditions*. These *conditions* are then treated with medications, often with disastrous results.

Do you know that 81% of our population is dying from either a chronic illness or man-made disease? Below are quotes from an article in the "Journal of the American Medical Association" (JAMA) that examined the causes of death over the last 100 years.

- This is the "age of degenerative and man-made diseases."

- "Chronic and neoplastic diseases account for 81.0% of deaths.[1]

Neoplastic diseases are tumors, and a neoplasm can be benign, potentially malignant (pre-cancer), or malignant (cancer).

So we have to ask: "What is causing these neoplasms and man-made diseases?" The answer lies in how we treat our health and how we treat our illnesses. The medical system is focused on a *symptom = drug protocol* that ignores the cause of the disease.

Imagine if disease didn't exist, and that disease is actually the body adapting to environmental influences. Imagine if Depression, Anxiety, High Blood Pressure, Fibromyalgia, Reflux, Irritable Bowel Syndrome, High Cholesterol, Crohn's

[1] Gregory L. Armstrong, MD; Laura A. Conn, MPH; Robert W. Pinner, MD. Trends in Infectious Disease Mortality in the United States During the 20th Century. *JAMA*. 1999; 281(1):61-66. doi:10.1001/jama.281.1.61.

Disease, Diabetes Type 2, and Attention Deficit Disorder, all came from the same source, i.e., an intelligent response of the body to toxicity and/or deficiency.

This book is dedicated to those people who have changed their perception of what health is and what disease is. If you change your perception, you change your world. If your perception is that you have a "disease or condition," you will treat that "disease or condition." If you change your perception about "disease" to disease being an intelligent response of your body adapting to toxicity or deficiency, you will then appreciate your body's response and recover health by correcting the deficiencies and eliminating the toxicities.

A total of 97% of all diseases come from either toxicity or deficiencies, but the medical cartel doesn't look into the results of a toxic or deficient lifestyle. In fact, the medications that are prescribed add to the toxic responses of the body. Just look at the *effects* of medications, which are called "side effects." They are actually not side effects; they are *effects*.

There are many doctors and many patients who have broken away from this "symptom drug protocol" and are looking at how to restore the natural state of health. Those revolutionaries (both doctors and patients) who have the idea that the body is a brilliant design and that health is the natural state of the body will change our world. In this book, I have included several of my patients as case studies. These are real people, just like you and me. I have changed their names, but all other information about them is completely accurate.

Scan this QR code for a video version of the highlights of this book.
Enjoy!

http://0s4.com/r/54J0OG

# Contents

## Disclaimer

You must not rely on the information in this book and/or video series as an alternative to medical advice from your doctor or other professional healthcare provider. If you have any specific questions about any medical matter, you should consult your doctor or other professional healthcare provider.

If you think you may be suffering from any medical condition, you should seek immediate medical attention. You should never delay seeking medical advice, disregard medical advice, or discontinue medical treatment because of information in this book and/or video series. Any change in medication, diet, and/or exercise should be directed by a qualified health care provider.

## Thanks and Appreciation

I wish to recognize my sons Michael and Danny who continue to inspire me with their courage in going against the norms of the status quo. Living healthy lifestyles and taking large bites out of life. I love you guys!

I also must express my appreciation for my daughter-in-law Karolina who is absolutely my son's soul mate. When she was diagnosed with hepatitis C, she became depressed. She then met my son, who made her aware of the miracle recovery her body was capable of. Through her trust and faith in my son's advice and natural therapies, she has recovered from Hepatitis C and depression. She now leads an active healthy lifestyle with limitless potential.

## Dedication

I am dedicating this book to Sarah, a patient of mine who demonstrated tremendous courage in taking charge of her own health. Diagnosed with depression and anxiety, and given multiple medications that left her with a miserable life, she was barely able to get out of bed. She was devastated, but the medical system could only offer her more powerful prescriptions with even more side effects. Finding strength within herself, and realizing that health was her natural state, she took charge of her mind and body as well as followed some simple steps to regain her life. She eliminated multiple medications; got her nervous system working correctly; changed her nutrition, which changed how her brain produced the chemicals that are emotions; and regained her life. She literally changed the structure of her brain using the techniques found in this book!

God bless you, Sarah.

Scan this QR code for a video version of the highlights of this book.
Enjoy!

http://0s4.com/r/54J0OG

# Chapter 1

## *Depression-/-Bipolar Disorder*
### *The Man-made Epidemic*

In this book we will explore some of the causes of and solutions to depression and bipolar disorder, but you have to know that the main cause has to do with digestion and how your brain reacts to stimulus, and the solution lies in understanding how your body works. I know that sounds weird, but when you look at this epidemic of mental disorders, you have to look at the causes.

Robert Whitaker wrote a brilliant book: *Anatomy of an Epidemic: Psychiatric Drugs and the Astonishing Rise of Mental Illness in America.*

One out of three Americans has some type of mental disorder! This is a problem of epic proportions.

If one out of three Americans has some type of mental disorder, the reality is that one in four women is taking some kind of medication for depression, anxiety and/or bipolar disorder. There is something wrong when 30% of a population has a disease or medical condition; there is a problem that needs a solution, not another medication. As an example: imagine if a herd of water buffalos had a third of their population running into trees or not being able to interact socially; would we treat that herd of water buffalos with medications or would we figure out the nature of the problem?

If you understand anatomy and physiology, the medical approach to depression, anxiety and bipolar disorder sounds completely insane. We are going to explore the most commonly ignored cause of these disorders. In the old days, and this is before the modern psychotropic anti-depressant drugs, patients diagnosed with severe depression would have to be hospitalized for it. Depression was considered short-term, six months hospitalization at most, and it was a one-time occurrence. So it was of short duration, people recovered and it typically never returned.

Before the era of modern antidepressant medications, bipolar disorder was extremely rare; it was almost unheard of. The current most popular therapy for depression/bipolar disorder is psychotropic medications, and if you're put on an antidepressant for five years, you have up to a 50% chance of being diagnosed as bipolar. Let's look at the antidepressants....

Take Prozac®, one of the most popular antidepressants. Does anybody know how Prozac works? If you have seen the advertisements or the commercials for antidepressant medications, what they advertise is a lie. The commercials show a young person running through a flowery field, happy and enjoying life. Then the announcer says it's "a selective serotonin reuptake inhibitor," which means there's something about serotonin that has to do with feeling good.

The problem is, when you look at the clinical *pharmacology,* or how the drugs actually work in your body (and this includes Prozac®, Depakote®, Wellbutrin®, Elavil®, and most of the antidepressants) what does it say? A quote from the package insert for Prozac® states: "**The mechanism of action of Prozac is unknown.**" That means that the doctors who prescribe these medications *don't know* how they work. How could you possibly call this science or accurate medical care? What's more, most of these types of medications have been studied for *only* 13 weeks before they are approved.

This means in regards to antidepressants, the doctors that prescribe them don't know how they work, and these drugs were approved with no studies existing longer than 13 weeks. Though doctors don't know how these drugs work, they do know some of the *effects* they have on patients. In pharmacology, these are called "side-effects." Here are some of the so-called "side-effects" of these medications, more accurately called "effects":

**Body as a Whole** — chills, suicide attempt, acute abdominal syndrome, photosensitivity reaction.

**Cardiovascular System** — palpitation, arrhythmia.

**Digestive System** — dysphagia, gastritis, gastroenteritis, melena, stomach ulcer, bloody diarrhea, ulcer esophageal ulcer, gastrointestinal hemorrhage, hematemesis, hepatitis, peptic ulcer, stomach ulcer hemorrhage.

**Hemic and Lymphatic System** — ecchymosis, petechia, purpura.

**Nervous System** — emotional liability, akathisia, ataxia, buccoglossal syndrome, euphoria, hypertonia, decreased libido, myoclonus, paranoid reaction, delusions.

**Respiratory System** — larynx edema.

**Skin and Appendages** — purpuric rash.

**Special Senses** — taste perversion, mydriasis.

These are just some the effects of the medications given to people who are depressed or sad or have anxiety.

Following is the Black Box warning placed on Prozac, a medication for depression and anxiety. (The Black Box warning is one of the strongest warnings that the FDA (Food and Drug Administration) can place on a medication.)

**WARNING:**

**SUICIDALITY AND ANTIDEPRESSANT DRUGS**

**Antidepressants increased the risk compared to placebo of suicidal thinking and behavior (suicidality) in children, adolescents, and young adults in short-term studies of Major Depressive Disorder (MDD) and other psychiatric disorders. Anyone considering the use of PROZAC or any other antidepressant in a child, adolescent, or young adult must balance this risk with the clinical need.**

Since the possible effects of this drug are suicidal thoughts and behavior, let's think about whom this drug is prescribed for: someone who is depressed and/or sad and/or anxious. The question that needs to be asked is: "Why is the symptom there?" or "What caused this depression/bipolar disorder?"

Let's look at some of the other "effects" of this medication like gastritis and emotional liability. These are major symptoms and they actually affect the root cause of this disorder. Look at the Prozac Black Box warning, then look at the Hippocratic Oath –

the oath that the doctors who prescribe these types of medications take in order to become "health care professionals."

**The Hippocratic Oath** states:

"I will use those dietary regimens which will benefit my patients according to my greatest ability and judgment, and I will do no harm or injustice to them.

"I will not give a lethal drug to anyone if I am asked, nor will I advise such a plan; and similarly I will not give a woman a peccary to cause an abortion."

Looking at that oath, how can a person who has taken the oath prescribe a drug that can cause **"suicidal thinking and behavior (suicidality) in children, adolescents, and young adults"**?

Doctors in Hippocrates' time, a few thousand years ago, practiced many unscientific, unsubstantiated therapies that were probably harming a lot of people. And that sounds like a lot of the medical therapies of today.

When you look at the actual warning on Prozac, this is the class of drugs used to treat depression. To give someone a drug that can cause: "increase the risk compared to placebos of suicidal thinking and behavior." Do you know what "suicidal behavior" is? It means trying to kill yourself!

This is a class of drugs that is supposed to effect serotonin levels.  What most people and doctors don't appreciate is that 90% of the body's serotonin is produced in *the gut*. That means that if there is less serotonin in the body effecting emotional health, there must be *a gut issue*.

The medical doctors that prescribe these drugs know that these antidepressants supposedly do something with serotonin. Are psychiatrists or medical doctors taught anything about nutrition or where serotonin is produced in the body? Unfortunately, the medical education in this country (U.S.A.) is lacking in natural causes and cures. The medical schools are funded by the Pharmaceutical industry, so the education of medical doctors is focused on a pharmaceutical approach that ignores, solution oriented, natural, non-toxic therapies.

# Chapter 2

## *Serotonin and How You Make It!*

The doctors of today are not taught about the many toxins that can negatively affect the natural serotonin production of the body. Let's look at serotonin and what it does, how it is produced, and what causes serotonin deficiencies.

If your serotonin is low, it can affect your:

- ✖ Mood

- ✖ Memory

- ✖ Ability to learn

- ✖ Appetite

- ✖ Arousal

- ✖ Aggression

- ✖ Impulse control

- ✖ Sexual desire

- ✖ Sleep

- ✖ Some social behaviors

- ✖ Heart

✖ Muscles

✖ Endocrine system (hormones)

Since up to 90% of serotonin production takes place in the gut, this means that gastric problems can cause all of the above issues. In turn, this means that Alzheimer's, dementia, mood problems, attention deficit disorder, depression, anxiety, arousal, (ED) erectile dysfunction, lack of desire, and impulse control can all be a problem of the digestive tract.

How many teenagers that have improper gut function also have impulse control issues? To find the solution symptoms, we need to look at the gut dysfunction that caused the symptoms.

To change the medical cartel's hold on the health care system, we need to look at history. You may have heard of the ancient medical procedure of "bleeding." Bleeding is the medical procedure that killed George Washington, our first president. Bleeding, first started by the Egyptians, was practiced for thousands of years. The theory behind "bleeding" was that disease was caused by "bad blood" or "evil spirits." The health care professionals would cut a vein and drain the bad blood off to get rid of the evil spirits or toxic blood. Let's look at history during the Black Plague in the Dark Ages when the wealthy died at greater rates than the poor. One theory is that the wealthy got the best medical care available at the time. If you had good medical care, during the dark ages, then you got a bleeding; and if you had really good medical care you got a bleeding *and* quicksilver. Quicksilver is mercury, and mercury is a powerful neurotoxin, meaning it is poison to the nervous system. In the past, mercury was prescribed for many conditions – from syphilis to common infections – and the joke of the time was "when you go to a medical doctor, all they ever do is give you quicksilver for everything. In fact, the practice of prescribing quicksilver was where we got the term "quack."

What is crazy is that modern psychiatry's drug therapies are based on supposed problems with brain chemistry or some type of mental dysfunction. Modern psychiatry has no "cures" for depression or anxiety; they just prescribe toxic drugs and thus change the symptoms.

For the cause and solution to depression and anxiety, we have to look to the cause. Since 90% of serotonin is produced in the *gut*, one of the causes of, and one of the solutions to, depression and anxiety lie in restoring healthy gut function and correcting any digestion problem. The most commonly overlooked cause of depression and anxiety is gut dysfunctions. Let's Heal Your Gut!

# Chapter 3

## *The Anatomy of Depression / Bipolar Disorder*

Digestion starts with smelling. Smelling stimulates the brain to cause acid secretions in your stomach. Then your saliva begins the digestion of carbohydrates, proteins are digested in the stomach and fats are digested in the intestines. So this beautiful process of digestion is the process of breaking down proteins to amino acids, fats to fatty acids, and carbohydrates to usable sugars. As for basic anatomy, you have a mouth that connects to a food tube called the esophagus. The esophagus leads to the stomach. The stomach leads to the small intestine and this is where most nutrients are absorbed. The small intestine is also where serotonin is produced, and anything that can damage the small intestine can effect serotonin production. In turn, anything that effects serotonin production will cause a host of symptoms, including depression, anxiety, and attention deficit disorder, just to mention a few. The intestinal tract looks just like a tube, but inside of this tube are structures called villi.

Villi look like fur covering the intestinal tract. These tiny villi are in the intestines to increase the surface area for your digestive process; you need a massive amount of surface area to complete the digestive process. Remember, you need to break proteins down to amino acids, and fats down to fatty acids, and carbohydrates down to usable sugars. That's the whole process of digestion. The amino acids, fatty acids and sugars are vital for tissue repair and life, and any problem with digestion will lead to deficiencies.

If you can't break down these proteins, fats, and/or carbohydrates, you end up deficient in vital nutrients that you need for every tissue and every process in your human body, including disease resistance and general health.

When people age, they wrinkle. When your skin wrinkles, it means that you can't break down proteins as well as you could when you were younger, or you're missing amino acids which is the basic building product for a healthy body. You might also be missing the enzymes that you need to break those proteins down to the amino acids, or you have some other type of stress on your digestion. We can take supplements or vitamins to compensate for these deficiencies. We can also juice or blend our food as this predigests the food and that can compensate for our lack of acid production as we age.

There is another problem that is often overlooked or not even recognized by the medical cartel of today, and that problem is "leaky gut." Leaky gut is a condition that causes undigested proteins to be leaked into the bloodstream. When your intestinal tract is working correctly, only digested materials pass through the wall of the intestines. Then the digested materials travel in a system of veins that drain into the liver to further complete digestion. I want you to appreciate how dynamic you truly are! You build *one billion cells a day* and you get the material to build those cells from your diet…so anything that is introduced into your diet literally becomes *you*. The main causes of depression and altered mental function, as well as most diseases, begin in the *gut*. Anything that damages these villi of the intestines, or anything that injures your digestion, can cause altered brain function. There are many chemicals and medications that we are exposed to today that can literally create *holes* in the intestines. If you have holes in your intestinal tract, this is called *leaky gut*, and it allows large undigested proteins to get into the bloodstream. As noted, the whole process of digestion is to break down the proteins to amino acids, the fats to fatty acids, and the carbohydrates to usable sugars; and the process of having large, undigested proteins in the bloodstream can cause an allergic reaction.

# Chapter 4

## *Allergic Reaction: A Missed Cause of Depression / Bipolar Disorder*

An allergy is an abnormal response to protein. You are built with a beautiful and strong immune system that is designed to identify abnormal proteins and attack them to protect your health. Viruses and bacteria are made of *proteins*, so an immune system response to these proteins keeps you alive. However, an allergy is an abnormal response; it is an over-reaction of your immune system to a foreign protein. That's *all* it is. Ask yourself: is hay fever caused by pollen? Nope, it's not, because I breathe pollen and I don't get an allergic response. So pollen can only cause hay fever or a problem if your body thinks that pollen is a pathogen. Sometimes the immune system can malfunction so badly that these hypersensitive reactions can even kill you. You have all heard of someone dying from a bee sting, or having a life-threatening episode from eating nuts. Those reactions are the body's abnormal recognition of those proteins. There's a really amazing mother by the name of Robyn O'Brien who has done research in this area and written a book. It's called *The Unhealthy Truth*. She was driven to write this book because of an event that almost cost the life of her child. She was serving breakfast to her four kids, a breakfast of waffles, yogurt, and eggs, and one of her children turned blue and almost died! It turned out that her child had had a severe allergic reaction to something in the food. So she's thinking, when did food become poisonous?

She wanted to find out the cause of this abnormal reaction. In fact, her child had an abnormal recognition of protein and that is what an allergic reaction is. What happens is, if the intestine has holes in it, undigested proteins can get into the bloodstream. So anything that creates holes in your intestinal tract, can cause abnormal digestion. And abnormal digestion can cause irritable bowel syndrome, Crohn's Disease, depression, and altered brain function from abnormal serotonin production.

# Chapter 5

## *Leaky Gut: Another Cause of Depression/Bipolar Disorder*

One of the most common and overlooked causes of attention deficit disorder, depression, anxiety, and bipolar disorder, can stem from a gut dysfunction. So many symptoms and health issues stem from the quality of food you put into your digestive system. If large undigested proteins pierce the gut – proteins such as caseins from toxic hormone-laden homogenized and pasteurized dairy, or glutens from genetically-modified wheat – they can actually attach to areas of your brain. Your brain has opiate receptors or pleasure sensors in the brain, and these large proteins can attach to those cells of the brain – which can actually starve the brain of nutrients.

Leaky gut is indicated in Alzheimer's, Dementia, Attention Deficit Disorder (ADD), Attention Deficit Hyperactivity Disorder (ADHD), and multiple other diagnoses. Our intestinal tract has evolved over 40,000 years, with complex chemical reactions that turn food into a human body. You not only are what you eat you actually, become what you eat.

The question needs to be asked: "Why is our brilliantly evolved digestive system starting to break down?" Well, first of all, there are unusual proteins in our food supply that we as a species have never been exposed to. Genetically Modified Organisms

(GMO's) have been introduced into our food supply beginning in 1996. These are seeds developed by a chemical company in order to sell more chemicals. GMO's are advertised as one of the greatest scientific breakthroughs of our time – a triumph of science over nature. In reality, GMO's are made by artificially inserting foreign genes into plants and animals. The theory is that for every gene there is a protein produced. So if you want a specific protein that may make a tomato more frost resistant, you just insert a gene from a cold-water fish. In theory, your tomato should then better withstand the cold weather. In fact, genes don't work that way; a human produces over 100,000 proteins, but we have slightly over 24,000 genes, a fruit fly has about 14,000. The science of modifying the genes of our food supply is fatally flawed. We now have unusual foreign proteins in our food, proteins that have never been tested in human beings. That is a tragedy. We need to ask the question: "Who would vote to put untested genetically modified materials in our food supply?" In America, the introduction of these GMO's was approved by a federal agency, the FDA (Food and Drug Administration). The FDA reasoned that these untested (in humans) Genetically Modified proteins haven't been proven dangerous, so they were given the label "G.R.A.S." (Generally Recognized As Safe). But they have never been proven to be safe!!!

Most of the world doesn't allow this genetically modified food unlabeled in their food supply. The U.S.A. cannot sell many of their food products in over 27 different countries because of the toxicity from the modified and untested genes. GMO's are banned in many countries in Europe, and one of the reasons these GMO's are banned is because they haven't been proven *safe*. Yet in the U.S.A., GMO's are allowed in our food supply because they haven't been proven *dangerous*. There have been no human studies conducted for GMO foods, in most of Europe they are either banned or at least labeled. There *have* been animal studies. The animal studies that have been done show that GMO's cause infertility in addition to a host of other ailments, including immune system problems, depression, accelerated aging, and the interruption of cholesterol synthesis or how you make cholesterol. Cholesterol is the main material your brain uses and most of your hormones plus cholesterol is vital for a healthy immune system. If you interrupt cholesterol synthesis, you're talking mental disorders, cancers, depression, and poor insulin regulation that can lead to diabetes. Then there are alterations in kidney, spleen, and gut function, all the result of introducing GMO's in our food supply. If you alter gut function, which is where serotonin is produced, you alter serotonin production. And altering serotonin production will absolutely affect the increase in incidence of a host of ailments, and diseases including depression, bipolar disorder and anxiety.

Given the effects of GMO's in our food supply, there have been several ballot measures by concerned organizations (including some U.S. states) trying to mandate the labeling of GMO foods.

What the average person needs to know is that, in the U.S.A., over 90% of the wheat, 95% of the soy products, and virtually every type of corn product in our food supply is genetically modified. So you should not eat those foods, unless they are labeled "organic." Organic foods have no GMO ingredients.

In 1992, the Food and Drug Administration (FDA) made this policy statement: "The agency is not aware of any information showing that foods derived from these new methods differ from any other foods in any meaningful or uniform way."

If you're not going to *look for* problems with GMO's, you're not going to *find* problems with GMO's. Remember, there are no human studies for GMO's unless you look at the current health of the American population. Look at the health of your family, friends and coworkers and you will see the result of this GMO human experiment. There is no doubt that the health of our population is rapidly deteriorating.

No part of the process of allowing untested GMO foods in our food supply makes sense. When you look at the studies of rats that are fed GMO foods, they show all kind of problems – from autism to reproductive issues to liver problems and altered physiology.

If you give rats a choice between genetically modified corn and not genetically modified corn, the rats will not eat the genetically modified corn, because the corn itself actually has pollen on it and the pollen is a neurotoxin. That is correct: a popular type of GMO corn was actually created to have pollen that killed insects. So the rats are smarter than we are. *The bottom line is that the GMO seeds are manufactured by a chemical company so they can sell more chemicals; they are not made for the health of our population.*

## Chapter 6

### *Nerve Poisons You Eat: Another Missed Cause*

Russell Blaylock wrote the book *Excitotoxins, the Taste That Kills*. If we're talking about depression and anxiety, excitotoxins are the most wonderful invention the world has ever seen (if you are a food manufacturer and not a consumer).

These excitotoxins are brilliant and amazing – if you have no ethics or morals. Let's look at one excitotoxin in particular; it's called MSG or monosodium glutamate. These nerve poisons attach to the pleasure centers in the brain and stimulate those centers. So I could take a sick, decayed, rotted piece of animal flesh that's actually putrid and I could roll it in genetically modified grain, freeze it, deep fry it in genetically modified hydrolyzed vegetable oil, and serve it to you. If I mix in MSG, kids will go crazy over it; we could call it chicken nuggets. If you serve this toxic food with a sauce that has even more neurotoxins, your taste buds will crave this potent brain toxin. If food contains MSG, which attaches to the pleasure sensors, it has a neurological effect; it affects brain function. This is the same effect that happens with the artificial sweeteners that are so popular in our food supply, like aspartame or nutrasweet®. When you are buying food and you are educated in the effects of the toxic food products that may be in processed foods, you will read the package labels looking for toxins like MSG. If MSG or aspartame or nutrasweet® or other toxins are on the food label, it means this food product can cause brain damage, learning disabilities, attention deficit disorder, depression, and bipolar disorders. The sweetener that is in Diet Coke® is chlorinated sugar called Splenda®; this and a host of other food products that have been allowed in our food supply are toxic to humans. These are the diet products that many people are ingesting every day. What are the teenagers drinking? What are they eating?

It is understandable that we have violent behavior in schools, because there's a loss of impulse control, and impulse control is part of the frontal lobe function of the brain. The frontal lobe of the brain is commonly injured in leaky gut conditions from various toxins and foreign proteins. Gut function is directly involved in impulse control, and genetically modified foods, antibiotics, vaccinations, and other neurotoxins can actually blow holes in the gut, causing frontal lobe damage.

So knowing the current state of our food supply, it's understandable that *one third* of our population is diagnosed with some type of mental disorder.

# Chapter 7

## *More Neurotoxins and Vaccines*

In some circles there is a huge controversy regarding the medical procedure of vaccination, which may cause harm and may not be good or appropriate for everyone. I'm not anti-vaccine, but I'm for effective healthcare procedures that are proven safe and effective. With all health care procedures there may be risks and may be benefits. This is called the risk/benefit ratio. For example, if a vaccine decreases measles in a certain portion of our population but causes autism in another segment of our population, then you have to weigh the damage of the disease versus the damage of the therapy. The science is there, proving that some vaccines can cause autism, brain damage, and a host of autoimmune disease. And some package inserts of vaccines list autism as a possible effect of the vaccine. However, vaccination still remains a main pillar of the medical cartel's protocols. The medical procedure of vaccination is rarely studied long term and *never* studied with the multiple dosages that are recommended by most medical doctors. This may come as a shock to the public to find out that a medical procedure that is recommended by nearly every health care professional is not based on scientific studies. The medical cartel holds the party line that vaccinations are based in science and they have "wiped out polio and small pox." That is the mantra that is repeated over and over by the medical profession. Here are some studies that show that vaccines may have contributed to epidemics like polio and autoimmune diseases:

**"Researchers have known since the early 1900s that paralytic poliomyelitis often started at the site of an injection. When diphtheria and pertussis vaccines were introduced in the 1940s, cases of paralytic poliomyelitis skyrocketed."** *Lancet* 1949

**Children who received DPT (diphtheria, tetanus, and pertussis) injections were significantly more likely than controls to suffer paralytic poliomyelitis within the next 30 days. According to the authors, "this study confirms that injections are an important cause of provocative poliomyelitis."** *Journal of Infectious Diseases* 1992

**"Even though the data regarding the relation between vaccination and autoimmune disease is conflicting, some autoimmune phenomena are clearly related to immunization."** J. Autoimmun. 2000 feb 14(1) 1-10.

A great book I recommend regarding the truth behind vaccinations is "Dissolving Illusions" by Dr. Suzanne Humphries M.D.

When you study the medical procedure of vaccination and the risk/benefit ratio for our population, the risks far outweigh any perceived benefit. The main benefit is financial – for our government (which holds patents on many vaccines) and for the pharmaceutical industry that manufactures them. The vaccine injury compensation program in America is evidence that there are risks to this medical procedure. The contents of the vaccines are not studied long term or individually, regarding how they may affect the person injected.

Here are some of the contents of the most used vaccines:

Vaccines may contain foreign DNA from insect cells, yeast, mouse brains, and tissue from pigs, guinea pigs, rabbits, dogs, calf lymph, hens' eggs, chick embryos, monkey kidney and testicle cells, retinal cells, aborted human fetal tissue, and cancer cells.

Then there are the preservatives used in some of the vaccines:

**Measles and Mumps Live Virus Vaccine**: (M-M-Rvax) Made by Merck. Contains gelatin, sorbitol, sodium chloride, bovine cow serum, and human albumin.

**Diptheria, Tetanus and Polio Vaccine:** Five injections given between two and six years of age, plus boosters "recommended" every 10 years. This vaccine contains formaldehyde, phenoxyethanol and aluminum phosphate.

**DTaP, IPV, HBV and Hib:** (Diphtheria, tetanus, polio, hepatitis B and Haemophilus influenza type B) Given to infants from two to 12 months old with boosters less than a year later; contains aluminum hydroxide, formaldehyde, and bovine cow serum.

MSG is just one of the ingredients used in vaccines. Some of the ingredients in vaccines are known neurotoxins, and there are also those animal proteins present in this medical procedure.

Remember what causes allergies: *allergies are the body's recognition of abnormal proteins.* Any medical procedure that introduces foreign proteins into the body can cause an allergic response from your immune system. There are many toxins today that people throughout history have never been exposed to. This toxic exposure has caused us to be one of the sickest populations in history with more cancers and chronic disease than have ever been seen previously. Here are some statistics and articles on the state of health of American children:

**2007 issue of Academic Pediatrics:** An estimated 43% to 54.1% of U.S. children (32 million) have a chronic health condition.

**2011 issue of Pediatrics:** Between 1997 and 2008, the number of school-age children diagnosed with autism, ADHD, or another developmental disability has risen 17%.

**2011 Archives of General Psychiatry:** and it found that the U.S. has the highest in the world lifetime rate of bipolar disorder at 4.4%

**2013:** Autism, ADHD, or another developmental disability=*amount to 21%* of children in the U.S.A.

It is time to take back our health by respecting that health is the natural state of the body. The health statistics of our population need to be a *wake-up call* because if the path we are on continues, more people will be sick than healthy. There needs to be *a health revolution!* And it's starting to happen: more people every day are questioning medical procedures like vaccinations and prescription drugs. Begin by asking your doctor what is broken in your body that is requiring this drug or medical procedure. Ask: "Why is this drug or medical procedure necessary?" Find out what are the long term effects of the medical procedure or drug. When you begin to ask those vital questions, you may find out that you are being prescribed medications that you do not need. Look at people choosing to not vaccinate their children; they are choosing a healthier lifestyle and better ways to strengthen the immune system. This revolution has to happen from the grass roots up. The current system of sick care is making too much money and has too much political power; at this point those in charge will not choose to change, so it is up to us to work toward change. The power needs to be in the hands of the people. Through education, our people, and I mean the people of the world, will take back their health.

Vaccinations, medications, and our food supply need to be examined in terms of how they affect the long term health of our bodies. Our planet will begin to change when people hold to the truths that *health is the natural state of the body* and "symptoms" are there for a reason. Treating symptoms may be the norm today, but this approach ignores the fact that symptoms are giving us a messages that will help to guide us back to health.

# Chapter 8

## *The Perfect Storm For Disease and Illness*

The genetically modified proteins in our diet, and the foreign proteins and toxins in our vaccines, and our over-medicated population make for the "perfect storm" of disease and illness. The viruses in a vaccine need to grow in living tissue, they are grown in cells and proteins from either animal flesh, human tissues, or yeasts. These viruses are all foreign proteins that are injected into the human body in the medical procedure called "vaccination," with dozens and dozens of vaccines currently recommended in a one-size-fits-all policy. Ask yourself: if 10 people all take the same drug, will they all have the same reaction? Of course not! Now translate that into tens of millions of children receiving all of those foreign proteins and neurotoxins – are they all going to have the same response? Now ask yourself the really hard questions, like: "Are there healthier ways to help an immune system, ways that are not toxic, like healthy food and vitamins and minerals?" We do have the power to take back our health!! Join this revolution!!

Before 1986, there were three vaccine manufacturers. Then our government passed a law stating that no vaccine manufacturer is liable for any damage that their products do; it is called the **"The National Childhood Vaccine Injury Act of 1986."** This law laid down the new rule that anyone injured by vaccination would be compensated by tax dollars and not by the companies or doctors responsible for the injuries. This law is kind of brilliant; I mean if you have no ethics or morals, you would appreciate it. A chemical company can produce a vaccine loaded with materials that can cause disease and injury and they are not responsible. This law opened up the lure of massive profits without risk, and the profits of chemical or pharmaceutical companies soared. Before our government passed these laws stating that the vaccine manufacturers are not liable, and that doctors are not liable for the medical procedure of vaccination, they were responsible for what they did. But now if a doctor injects your child or you with a vaccine and this causes autism, or attention deficit disorder, or cancer, or Guillain-Barre, or paralysis, you cannot sue for damages as long as the vaccine is on *the recommended schedule*. So what does that mean? When this new law was passed, any vaccine that was added to *the recommended schedule* was protected from financial liability. Under this law, when a pharmaceutical company sells a vaccine, they are liable for it *unless* it is on *the recommended schedule*. So guess what was added to the recommended vaccine schedule? The flu shot, and dozens of other vaccines. Just look at the Hepatitis B vaccine. Hepatitis B is common in IV drug users and sexually active people; infants are not at risk for it. But it was put on the recommended schedule so no one but the taxpayers were liable. Think about that risk/benefit ratio when looking at infants and Hepatitis B. That is why the "recommended" vaccine schedule went from 10 vaccines in 1986 to *38 vaccines before the age of 6 years old* in 2014! And did our population get healthier? No. In fact, we have one of the sickest and most medicated populations the world has ever seen.

Now look at how they measure if a vaccine is effective. Of course you can't give a vaccine and then throw buckets of Hepatitis on someone and say, "Well, he didn't get sick so the vaccine must have protected him." You can't do that. It doesn't work that way, because if everybody's exposed to a virus, it doesn't mean everybody's going to get sick. We all have different immune systems. The way that is used to test if a vaccine is effective is to inject the vaccine and then test the antibodies that it produces.

Let's look into the Hepatitis B vaccine. If you look at the Center for Disease Control (CDC) website, it says that if you have greater than 10 antibodies per milliliter then you have sufficient protection from hepatitis. Now there's no actual science behind this number of 10 antibodies per milliliter; it is just a guess, because a person can have lots of antibodies for any given disease and still get the disease, and they can also have few antibodies for the disease and not get sick. Nevertheless, the CDC says that if you have greater than 10 antibodies per milliliter, you're protected. So let's just take that guess as science and look at some journal articles that examine the effects of the Hepatitis vaccine:

**2004 Journal of Neurology:** The Hepatitis B vaccine is associated with an increased risk of multiple sclerosis.

**2009 Journal of Lupus:** Vaccination is associated with a rare autoimmune neurological condition, transverse myelitis.

**2005 Journal of Autoimmunity:** Hepatitis B vaccination significantly increases the risk of a wide range of autoimmune diseases.

**2002 Journal of Clinical Rheumatol:** Adult rubella and adult hepatitis B vaccines were statistically associated with chronic arthritis which persisted for at least one year.

**2009 Journal of Clinical Nueromuscular Distrophy:** In the U.S., the highest number of cases of Guillian-Barre Syndrome are associated with the influenza and hepatitis B vaccine. J Clin Nueromuscul Dis. 2009 Sep; 11 (1): 1-6

**2010 Journal of Vaccine:** There were 69 reports of Guillian-Barre Syndrome (GBS) after Gardasil vaccination that occurred in the United States between 2006 and 2009.

Let's look at the antibody production from just one study following the injection of a group of infants, teens and adults:

Engerix-B Vaccine Study

|              | Amount  | Time      | Antibodies        |
|--------------|---------|-----------|-------------------|
| Adults:      | 20 ugm  | 7 months  | 2,2284 mIU/ml     |
|              | 20 ugm  | 13 months | 9,163 mIU/ml      |
| Adolescents: | 10 ugm  | 8 months  | 1,989mIU/ml       |
|              | 20 ugm  | 8 months  | 7,672 mIU/ml      |
| Infants:     | 10 ugm  | 4 months  | 2,942 mIU/ml      |
|              | 10 ugm  | 7 months  | 713 mIU/ ml       |

Now let's look at the adults: at 13 months after the injection, they got a 20 microgram of injection, they had 9163 units per milliliter of antibodies. Now that's nearly *1000 times* the amount of antibodies that the CDC says is necessary for protection from hepatitis B. So you have hundreds of times more of these antibodies floating around in your bloodstream with no virus to attack. The function of an antibody – and I want you to burn this into your soul, the function of an antibody is to *attach* to a virus or bacteria and start the immune system response to *kill* the pathogen.

So what happens to your health when you have thousands of times more antibodies floating around in your human body without any disease other than what was injected into you by this vaccination to form these antibodies? What about an infant who has an immature immune system? What about an adolescent who is also exposed to other environmental toxins?

Below are quotes from a medical journal linking vaccinations to various diseases caused by vaccine reactions:

- ✖ molecular mimicry is an important factor in autoimmune disease

- ✖ first published in 1985 and since that time substantial evidence has accumulated

- ✖ causing many autoimmune diseases including: **diabetes, lupus, scleroderma, rheumatoid arthritis, multiple sclerosis, chronic fatigue syndrome, autism**

- ✖ "…even though the data regarding the relation between vaccination and autoimmune disease is conflicting, some autoimmune phenomena are clearly related to immunization."

J. Autoimmun. 2000 feb 14(1) 1-10

The science is there: vaccines are linked to many of the diseases that are at an epidemic level in our population. And these vaccine policies will not be questioned because they are part of the infrastructure of our medical system. Changing the current system has to be done from the ground up. In the future it's not going to be 36 vaccines recommended for everyone; it's going to be more. More vaccines are being developed for infants, teens, and adults because of the extreme profitability for the pharmaceutical and medical industry. It's not about health at all; it's about money.

I'm for safe and effective health care procedures; I'm not in favor of subjecting our people and our children and our infants to experimental procedures. In the future, instead of vaccinating everyone regardless of their antibody levels, each person should be checked for their own antibody levels for each particular disease. No medical procedure should ever be a one-size-fits-all procedure without regard for the individual's immune system response. For example, it is possible that there could have been a natural exposure to a given disease and that your body has already developed natural immunity to that disease, so let's check antibody levels first. Wouldn't that make more sense? Now let's look at the connection between vaccinations, molecular mimicry and excess antibody production, and their link to depression, anxiety and bipolar disorders. When you look at how these antibodies are designed to attack certain proteins and pathogens, it's clear they can also attack the gut, damaging the gut. And these antibodies can attack other parts of the body as well. If they attack cartilage, you get diagnosed with rheumatoid arthritis. If they attack the pancreas, you get diagnosed with diabetes. If they attack the brain, you get autism or some other neurological disease. These excess antigens are injected into you, your kids, and our whole population – from the flu shot, from the Hepatitis B shot, from the diphtheria shot, etc. All of these vaccinations cause immune system responses that can have disastrous consequences. Vaccinations are linked to diseases like multiple sclerosis, autism, chronic fatigue, fibromyalgia and many more. This is in the science journals. It's not a guess. This is what's actually happening to the population of our country.

Remember this quote from the Journal of Autoimmune Disorders: "Even though the data regarding this relationship between vaccines and autoimmune disease is conflicting, some autoimmune phenomena are clearly related to immunizations."

When you add up the effect of vaccinations, medications, and our toxic food supply, you have a toxic overload that is destroying the health of our population. Here's a startling fact: children who eat three hot dogs a week have a ten to twelve time's higher risk of getting brain cancer or leukemia. That isn't a 10% or 12% higher risk; its *10 or 12 times* the risk. Why? Because they are ingesting abnormal proteins and other toxins that cause abnormal gut function and an altered immune system. Cancers don't come from bad luck or bad genes; they come from deficiency and toxicity.

Polio Vaccine

Last night I was watching a foreign news channel that has a different view of the news of the world than the popular news stations in the U.S.A. If you can, get cable, and look at different perspectives. It's very interesting what the rest of the world looks at. So they're talking about polio eradication in India, and they're showing this child sitting where sewage is running down the middle of the street. Polio is rampant in this area with 174 reported cases. Is there any wonder that diseases would be rampant in this area? Is polio infecting people because of lack of vaccinations, or is it because of lack of sanitation, unclean living conditions, poor nutrition, and stress? It is very expensive to fix the infrastructure and provide clean water and good sewage disposal and fresh food and refrigeration. So the cheaper solution is to shoot the population with vaccines.

Do vaccines protect a kid living in those squalid living conditions? When we look at this area, there were 174 cases of polio, and by 2010 it had dropped to only 42 cases. So if we get no more information, it seems that the vaccines are working, right? The 42 cases were reported as "wild polio." However, at the same time in the same area, there has been a massive epidemic of a devastating disease called "non-polio acute flaccid paralysis." This is from the vaccine, and it has all the symptoms of polio; but in the medical world, if you've been vaccinated you can't possibly have polio, so it must be something different. To find out if a person has polio, you have to check the stools. They're looking at these kids' stools to see if they can find "wild polio" and it's not there. Currently there are about 47,000 cases of acute non-polio flaccid paralysis and rising.

Some sources are reporting over 60,000 cases of acute non-polio flaccid paralysis from the vaccine, but out of those 60,000 kids with flaccid paralysis polio-like symptoms, only one of them tested positive for wild polio, so the vaccination program is a "success." Think of this: there are 60,000 kids that are paralyzed, and that are going to live the rest of their lives dysfunctional, but the polio program is considered successful, because only one of them tested positive for "wild polio." I encourage everyone to do further research and decide for themselves if injecting foreign proteins (vaccinations) is harmful or necessary. Carefully look into the risk/benefit ratio and make your decisions based on science, not on fear or hype. When it comes to medical procedures, it is not a one-size-fits-all process.

Autism

When we look at the epidemics that are currently plaguing our society, you can't ignore Autism. At this time, some estimates are as high as 1 in 25 boys. This diagnosis goes up about 10 to 12% a year, so it's 1 in 25 boys and climbing. The human being has never been assaulted with so many foreign proteins and neurotoxins, so this number will climb, thus contributing to the rise in stress and depression that we are also plagued with. *If there is no change in the increasing rate of autism, by 2026 the number of autistic kids will actually outnumber the kids without autism!* With regard to the massive increase in non-polio acute flaccid paralysis in India, a comment from a reader of the Hindustan Times asks a deep question: "I'm super-puzzled. There are over 60,000 cases of acute flaccid paralysis. This means that a huge number of children are paralyzed or partially paralyzed and will be struggling for the rest of their lives, and this is okay? As long as the paralysis is caused by something else, not polio?" The person has got common sense.

Depression and Anxiety

Another critical question is: what causes depression and anxiety – conditions that have become rampant in our society? It is clear that the cause is poisoning or altered gut function leading to altered brain function, as illustrated below.

**Case Study:** "Mary," a 38-year-old single mom with 2 children, 7 and 10 years old. She works at a stressful office job. She has neck pain, can't sleep well, her feet hurt occasionally, and she just feels not well. She goes to her medical doctor for help and he prescribes the antidepressant Prozac® to help her feel better, an anti-inflammatory for her feet, a sleep medication, and a pain reliever for her neck. Now she is taking four medications; is that going to upset her digestive tract? Okay, so she self-medicates with an over-the-counter antacid.

Luckily, a friend tells her that the medications she is taking are not making her healthy and have toxic side effects. Mary then came to our office looking for a solution. We did a complete exam and x-rays and found the source of her neck and foot pain, and we also identified abnormal gut function.

Mary was started on a plan to get her health back, and within 30 days she was drug-free, feeling great, sleeping well, and she even had her kids on her "new health kick."

It's so simple when you look at the body as constantly regenerating. The body has an innate intelligence, so your body will never give you a symptom unless there is a reason for the symptom. Your body always responds correctly to the stimulus given.

So did we fix Mary's gut? Did we get rid of her pain? No! What we did was correct the nerve pressure and remove the toxic stress load and her body healed itself. We corrected the *source* of her symptoms. Then we guided her in lifestyle adjustments to get back her vitality. Health is the natural state of the beautiful human body.

# Chapter 9

## *The Beauty of Your Autonomic Nervous System*

Here's a brief overview of your autonomic nervous system. It takes care of you automatically and it is composed of two parts. One part keeps you alive under stress and is called the "the fight-or-flight system" or the sympathetic nervous system. The other part is called "the rest, digest and repair system" or the parasympathetic system. When one system is activated, the other is essentially deactivated. Imagine that you are resting in an easy chair and all of a sudden an unexpected loud bang goes off, or you are driving and someone cuts you off in traffic, or you are doing a super workout at the gym. In any stressful circumstance, intentional or unintentional, your fight-or-flight system is activated. You can boil all stressors down to physical, chemical, or emotional causes. What is wild is that your body doesn't know the difference between physical, chemical or emotional stressors; it just kicks in this fight-or-flight system to keep you alive in the short term.

To protect you in the short term, this system raises your heart rate, reduces blood supply to the gut or digestion, decreases your immune system, and increases LDL cholesterol (this type of cholesterol is called "bad cholesterol" by some doctors who forget it has a major function, namely that it's used for tissue repair and is the precursor or building material for hormone production). So when the fight-or-flight system is engaged, people may be misdiagnosed with high blood pressure, high blood sugar, high cholesterol, digestive problems, depression, etc…. I say *misdiagnosed* because the underlying cause of the problem was not identified, appreciated or taken care of. To heal the cause of Depression/Bipolar disorder you have to have a healthy autonomic nervous system. What is interesting is that both parts of this nervous system are located in the brain and spinal cord. The Parasympathetic or "Rest, Digest, and Repair" system is located in the cranial and sacrum areas. The Sympathetic or "Fight or Flight" system is located in your thoracic and lumbar areas. Physical stress on the spine can cause stress on this nervous system. What is completely underappreciated is the day-to-day physical stress you are under. Imagine driving to work in stop-n-go traffic, then sitting at a desk for eight hours. Do you think this will cause tight shoulders and/or stress on your nervous system? That is why to recover from any disease, including Depression/Bipolar disorder, it is vital to balance your autonomic nervous system.

**Case Study:** Mike, a 48-year-old contractor happily married with three children. Mike came in with Erectile Dysfunction (ED), fatigue, sleep problems, depression, chronic tightness between his shoulders, and his hands would occasionally hurt. Mike was taking Tylenol®, medications for High Blood Pressure, Wellbutrin® (for anxiety), and Viagra® for his ED.

We did a complete exam including a Heart Rate Variability study, a surface Electro Myography study, and a digital x-ray. We found that the source of his hand pain and chronic tight shoulders was the pinched nerves in his neck caused by misaligned vertebrae or "subluxations." This was keeping him in a "fight or flight" mode causing his High Blood Pressure, and the High Blood Pressure medications were causing the Erectile Dysfunction.

We started immediately reducing pressure on his nervous system and his blood pressure normalized without medications within 2 weeks. His sleep patterns changed within 3 weeks, and after 8 weeks he had no more need for his Wellbutrin® (for anxiety) and Viagra® (for his ED). We didn't heal him; we just reduced the pressure on his nervous system, and that changed him from a sympathetic dominant system to a normally balanced nervous system. His body was responding correctly to stress when he had the High Blood Pressure and ED. The key to getting Mike's health back was: we didn't treat the symptoms; we respected his symptoms as an intelligent response of his body, and we corrected the cause allowing his body to heal itself.

# Chapter 10

## *The Body's Intelligent Response to Stress*

Here's an example: The current popular belief in health care is that there are four risk factors for heart disease: smoking, diabetes, high cholesterol, and high blood pressure. In my world, the body is self-regulating, so high cholesterol and High Blood Pressure are actually the body adapting to toxic circumstances. When you know that cholesterol is the building material for cortisol (an anti-inflammatory produced by your adrenal glands) and High Blood Pressure is an intelligent stress response, then two of the "four risk factors" are a clue to a body under stress.

Even type 2 diabetes is the body either generating excess energy because of stress, or a response to excess sugars or toxic fats; so type 2 Diabetes could be your body adapting to a toxic or deficient environment. For an example, let's look at the smoking diabetic that has high cholesterol and High Blood Pressure. So he has all four risk factors – did you know that less than 1.0% of everyone with heart disease has all four risk factors? So the truth is that at least two of those "four risk factors" are the body correctly adapting to the environment. They're not risk factors; they're clues to what the body is adapting to.

Here is a study linking low cholesterol to depression:

## Low Cholesterol Linked to Depression

Dutch researchers studied 30,000 men and found that low cholesterol levels meant an increased risk of depression in men. They found that men with chronically low cholesterol levels showed a consistently higher risk of having depressive symptoms along with anger, hostility, and impulsivity.

**Psychosomatic Medicine 2000; 62.**


Since 80% of your total cholesterol is produced by your body, and cholesterol is vital for hormone production and the main material the brain is made of, does it make sense that low cholesterol can cause a hormone imbalance and brain dysfunction?

Imagine you're being chased by a tiger – what would happen to your heart rate? Your heart rate would have to go up. Now do you want blood going to digestion or blood going to your arms and legs? You need more blood to your arms and legs to run away from danger, and you will sacrifice blood supply for digestion. So that means, under stress – whether physical, chemical, or emotional stress, as all three cause the same response in your body – your heart rate elevates, your blood supply to the gut shuts down, your blood sugar elevates. Where is serotonin produced? You remember that the feel-good hormone serotonin is produced in the gut! This means that chronic sympathetic stimulant, or chronic fight or flight, is eventually going to lead to abnormal gut function and abnormal serotonin production and lead to Depression/Bipolar Disorder along with a host of other symptoms.

Just think of what happens when you decrease digestion or when your gut function is altered by stress:

- you can't break down proteins to amino acids

- you can't break down fats to fatty acids

- you can't break down carbohydrates to usable sugars.

That's why in order to solve Depression/Bipolar Disorder, you've got to look at the nervous system first, then you look at the stress hormones, then you look at rewiring your brain.

Stress hormones are absolutely vital to keep you alive in the short term; however, they can also do damage to your system if your stress response remains activated.

# Chapter 11

## *Rewiring Your Brain*

Emotions are chemicals created by electrical signals from your brain based on your perceptions. Let me explain this in plain English. You interpret thoughts and environmental stimulus to be good/bad/joyous/fearful/loving/hateful, etc...based on how you perceive "it" to be. For an example: let's say you see a cute furry puppy. If you have fond memories of cuddling or petting a puppy in the past, your brain, using that past memory, will cause a set of chemicals to be released that will trigger the emotions of joy/love/happiness. However, if you have memories of being bitten by a cute puppy, your brain will use that past experience to secrete chemicals related to stress/fear/anger.

For another example: let's say you and I ride a roller coaster. You love roller coasters and at the end of the ride you are filled with joy; this comes from your brain causing the chemicals to be produced and creating the emotion of joy. Your whole body will respond with an increased immune response and a host of beneficial metabolic responses. On the other hand, let's say I have a fear of roller coasters, so at the end of the ride my metabolic response will be that of massive stress; cortisol and adrenaline will be flooding my body; and my immune system will be weakened. We had the same stimulus of the roller coaster ride, but based on our past memories, we had massively different responses. So in reality we are living in the past. Everything that happens to us, whether an event or thought or stimulus, we interpret according to how our brain is wired.

Your brain is composed of nerve cells that have connections called dendrites. These nerve cells connect the dendrites together by way of a synapse to hold your memories, thoughts, experiences, etc., and this is how the brain works. Imagine two trees with hundreds of branches and each branch making a connection with one or two branches of a neighboring tree, and now imagine a billion trees with a trillion connections. Then you have a small idea of how your brain works.
The human brain:
- has an estimated hundred billion neurons;
- has several hundred trillion synaptic connections;
- and can process and exchange prodigious amounts of information over a distributed neural network in a matter of milliseconds.

This is how the brain is wired together, and the nerve cells that are wired together fire together. So now we have a group of nerve cells that fire together, are wired together, produce consistent chemicals, and produce consistent emotions.

Think of a professional tennis player. Through practice, his brain will wire the physical responses required for quick hand and eye coordination, and he will also have to wire his perception to the stress of a professional tennis match. So his perception of facing a hundred-mile-an-hour tennis ball flying toward his head would be greatly different than that of the average person. His brain, through training, is now wired for this event, and his perception is altered based on how his brain is wired and how it fires.

For another example: look at someone famous, wealthy, successful, and depressed. We all have heard of stories in the news of a famous actor or sports hero that, despite having what most people would perceive as a wonderful life, has mastered depression. Now hold this thought, I know that when I say "mastered depression" I'm not making light of depression. I want you to appreciate that emotions are chemicals produced from how the brain cells are firing based on perception of the environmental stimulus.

A person sees a beautiful Rolls Royce and may perceive unnecessary luxury or waste of money. Those thoughts are the result of chemicals made from how your brain is wired. Another person would be excited and envious.

I want you to realize that how you view your personal reality is the *truth* to you. If you view yourself as happy, confident, healthy, successful, that is true for you. If you view yourself as depressed, shy, sick, sad, a failure, that is true for you. So how you view yourself, or what you think of as your personal reality, makes up your personality.

Let's free your potential! What if you could alter your personality and then change your personal reality! You are not a slave of your reality; you are a slave of your perception of your reality, and your perception can change. Think of this: if we can change your perception, we change how your brain cells fire;

and that changes the way your brain is wired; and that changes the chemicals produced; and that changes your emotional state!! Let's put you back in charge!! Here is a great article on "neuroplasticity" that means you can change your brain.

**Environment and brain plasticity:**
**towards an endogenous pharmacotherapy**
Physiol Rev. 2014 Jan

"Brain plasticity refers to the remarkable property of cerebral neurons to change their structure and function in response to experience
…how changes at the level of neuronal properties can ultimately affect and direct key perceptual and behavioral outputs.
…striking ability of environmental enrichment and physical exercise to empower adult brain plasticity."
This type of article gives me goose bumps; think of what endogenous pharmacotherapy means. It means that you can produce the chemicals you need to produce the emotions you want, on your own without any negative side effects. This means when you change your *perception*, you will produce the right "drug" in the right dosage at the right time without side effects and without a prescription!

# Chapter 12

## *Changing the Structures of the Brain*

Let's now look at some amazing aspects of how you can actually change the structures of the brain. Let's start with the hippocampus. It is part limbic system and it has some awesome functions:

- Incoming sensory signals are retransmitted and initiate behavioral reactions
- Pleasure
- Rage
- Passivity
- Excessive sexual drive
- **Modulation of emotions**
- **Involved in mood disorders, depression, bipolar disorder**

And in at least three different psychiatric conditions, there is shrinkage (atrophy) of the hippocampus:

**Depression**
**Post-Traumatic Stress Disorder**
**Bipolar Disorder**

Below is a great journal article on the structural changes that occur in the brains of people suffering from Depression/Bipolar Disorder:

### Hippocampal interneurons in bipolar disorder

Arch Gen Psychiatry. 2011; 68(4):340-50 (ISSN: 1538-3636)
(Hippocampus is smaller in people with bipolar disorder)

Another journal discusses how the hippocampus may be involved in the cause of bipolar disorder:

**The role of hippocampus in the pathophysiology of bipolar disorder.**
Behav Pharmacol. 2007 Sep;18(5-6):419-30.

"...the available evidence suggests that the hippocampus plays an important role in the pathophysiology of Bipolar Disorder."

So by now I hope you have a greater appreciation of the role of the brain and the hippocampus and perception in depression/bipolar disorder. Let's build that hippocampus and change our brains.

Here is a great article on how to physically change your hippocampus:

## Psychiatry Research: Neuroimaging
Volume 191, Issue 1, Pages 36-43, 30 January 2011

### Mindfulness practice leads to increases in regional brain gray matter density

"The results suggest that participation in Mindfulness-Based Stress Reduction (MBSR) is associated with changes in gray matter concentration in brain regions involved in learning and memory processes, emotion regulation, self-referential processing, and perspective taking."

MBSR is a combination of yoga and meditation, and exercise is a great way to build the gray matter and the hippocampus:

**Researchers at Harvard, Yale, and the M.I.T. first evidence that meditation can alter the physical structure of our brains**

"Our data suggest that meditation practice can promote cortical plasticity in adults in areas important for cognitive and emotional processing and well-being."

"These findings are consistent with other studies that demonstrated increased thickness of:
- music areas in the brains of musicians
- visual and motor areas in the brains of jugglers.

In other words, the structure of an adult brain can change in response to repeated practice."

This science-based research demonstrates that there is a structural problem in depression and bipolar disorder and that there are solutions. I want you to appreciate that you have the power to change how your brain is wired through exercise, meditation, and a change in your perception. This approach is far removed from making you a victim and giving you a toxic drug with disastrous side effects. Understand your brain is like a battery, and it gets its charge from the normal position and motion of your vertebrae. A huge factor in altered information to the brain is altered position of the spinal vertebrae.

To summarize this rewiring of your brain:

- your emotions are chemicals produced by the way your brain is wired now

- the structures of your brain can change in shape

- the structures of the brain can change how they are wired

- your emotions are based on your past perceptions

- your past perceptions are based on how your neurons fire together

- your neurons cause your body to produce the chemicals of emotions

- your emotions become your personal reality

- you have the ability to change your brain structure and wiring through mediation, movement, detoxing, and a healthy nervous system.

One of the most important aspects of rewiring your brain is your self-talk. How you communicate with yourself about yourself, or other people or situations, is important, and it is vital to take control of this conversation. Here are the exercises to rewire your brain and change your self-talk and also a video on self-talk:

https://www.youtube.com/watch?v=s0MYe25ro1o

A great rewiring exercise is to say out loud the list below at least 4 or 5 times a day for 21 days. If possible, look into a mirror when doing this exercise:

| | | |
|---|---|---|
| I am Enthusiastic Compassionate | I am Fulfilled | I am |
| I am Fascinated | I am Friendly | I am Interested |

| | | |
|---|---|---|
| I am Invigorated | I am Peaceful | I am Loving |
| I am Intrigued | I am Lively | I am Encouraged |
| I am Open-hearted | I am Passionate | I am Optimistic |
| I am Relaxed | I am Relaxed | I am Sympathetic |
| I am Stimulated | I am Vibrant | I am Amused |
| I am Satisfied | I am Delighted | I am Serene |
| I am Blissful | I am Glad | I am Empowered |
| I am Awed | I am Ecstatic | I am Happy |
| I am Tranquil | I am Open | I am Elated |
| I am Trusting | I am Proud | I am Safe |
| I am Amazed | I am Exuberant | I am Tickled |
| I am Enlivened | I am Secure | I am Animated |
| I am Radiant | I am Rejuvenated | I am Absorbed |
| I am Thrilled | I am Comfortable | I am Excited |

Saying the above list out loud actually rewires your brain to change your self-talk, and that is key to recovery from Depression/Bipolar disorder.

Here is another talk I gave on changing your thought pattern:

https://www.youtube.com/watch?v=6N2BLlKYwz8

There are also some techniques to deal with past trauma's that I like and recommend.

Here is the web site for the Emotional Freedom Technique or EFT: http://www.emofree.com/

There is also Eye Movement Desensitization and Reprocessing (EMDR). Below is a condensed version of how to do EMDR. (It is used by the military.)

*Emotions are held in the right brain; the left brain is the logic center. The goal is to shift the memory from the right brain to the left brain; that way the memory becomes just a memory.*

*Steps:*

1. *Write down the situation that you are going to work on (thoughts, feelings, emotions – be explicit).*

2. *Find yourself two points on an opposite wall about 8 to 10 feet apart (whatever you feel comfortable with).*

3. *Keep your eyes moving from right to left then left to right and say "I didn't deserve that (abuse, beating, treatment, rape). I'm a good person, it's not my fault...." Say all of the things you need to say. Then have your most compassionate adult self-talk to the kids (yourself at the time of the trauma) at whatever ages they are and tell them you will always protect them. You are their good parent and you will not allow anything to happen to them. When you feel a release in your body, you can stop moving your eyes back and forth.*

4. *Sometimes there is a little more left, and just with more questioning you will know what it is and you can deal with that... In abuse it is often that the mom knew and did nothing, and before the person can heal, they have to work on their own issue.*

5. *Anchoring after you have made certain there is no more of*

*that trauma…. Identify a word that exemplifies yourself, whether you are this word now or will be in the future. Just one word like…*

*Empowered, Confident, Courageous, Strong, Healthy, Vibrant, etc..*

*Then say the word and clap. Do this 3 times.*

By using the power word list daily, using EFT or EMDR if necessary, and following the information on the videos, you will have the keys to brain rewiring.

# Chapter 13

## *You Must Take Control of Your Genes*

To recover from Depression / Bipolar Disorder, changing your thoughts and changing your perception of these diseases are vital to your recovery. To heal, you must heal on the cellular level in order to change your brain. Let's break down a huge falsehood: Depression/Bipolar Disorder is NOT GENETIC!! There is a huge difference between genetic *disease* and genetic *expression*. Genetic expression is in your control and you must take control of your gene expression to recover from Depression/Bipolar Disorder. Many people, including many doctors, are under the impression that many diseases are genetic. The fact is that *less than three percent* of diseases are genetic in origin. Down's Syndrome is a good example of a genetic disease; people who are born with this disease have a gene defect. Blue eyes are a genetic condition as well; you don't suddenly wake up one morning and say. "Wow, my blue eyes have turned brown." That would be impossible. When people say "It runs in my family," that is genetic *expression*, not a genetic *condition*. The difference between a genetic disease and the genetic *expression* of a disease is: if a disease develops in your 20's, 30's, 40's, 50's, or later in life, that disease is the body copying a part of your DNA that will express a disease. Cancer, Diabetes, and Depression/Bipolar Disorder are not genetic diseases; even if your uncle, dad, and sister all developed cancer or diabetes or were diagnosed with bipolar disorder, you don't have to develop those diseases. In these cases, how we *express* genes is everything. By everything, I mean you can develop disease or reverse disease. The control of what genes you express is above the genes; in other words, it is "epigenetic" control. Your body is a collection of 70 trillion cells. Each cell has to take in nutrients, produce proteins, and eliminate waste products. The proteins that your cells produce are chosen from parts of your DNA. I want you to get how important the proteins are; how you produce these proteins will reverse disease or cause disease. The parts of DNA you *choose* to express are the key to health or disease.

Dr. Bruce Lipton said it best: *"DNA does not control our biology;* instead, DNA is controlled by signals from outside the cell, including the energetic messages emanating from our positive and negative thoughts."* Your awareness of the fact that health is your natural state is a vital step in recovery and in regaining your health and vitality. A great book to read is *"The Biology of Perception"* by Dr. Bruce Lipton. He covers how perception of the environment changes protein production. So it's not what is really happening to you; it's how you perceive the event. Perception translates to different DNA production, and that will make us resistant to disease or lead to disease. To recover from Depression/Bipolar Disorder, you have to change your perception and also change how your brain is wired and how it fires. Your pattern of perception alters DNA expression and alters the structures of your brain; and that alters the chemicals produced; and that alters your emotional state either causing disease or curing disease. This is where daily meditation, daily prayer, and/or visualization are vital for full recovery. It is also important to know that prescription medications can cause epigenetic changes, as noted in *Metabolism Clinical and Experimental* 57: (2008) S16–S23.

Drugs that are known to cause epigenetic changes include:

- statin cholesterol-lowering drugs
- antidepressants
- beta blockers
- diuretics
- tamoxifen
- methotrexate
- anti-inflammatories
- even anesthetics
- oral contraceptives
- antibiotics.

Look at the journal article below:

**Permanent Changes in the Epigenome**

Researchers are most concerned that drugs may produce defects in subsequent generations. They speculate that the current diabetes epidemic may be hastened by drugs.

"...FDA-approved pharmaceutical drugs can cause persistent epigenetic changes."

"...pharmaceuticals may be involved in the etiology of *heart disease, cancer, nerve and mental disorders, obesity, diabetes, leukemia, bipolar disorder, schizophrenia, infertility, and sexual dysfunction.*"

"...consequences for modern medicine are profound, since it would imply that our current understanding of pharmacology is an oversimplification."

*Metabolism Clinical and Experimental* 57: (2008) S16–S23.

Given the information above – that FDA-approved pharmaceutical drugs can cause persistent epigenetic changes – recovery from Depression/Bipolar Disorder *cannot* involve a pharmaceutical or medication approach. In fact, Depression/Bipolar Disorder may be worsened by many prescription medications and even caused by some. If you are taking prescription medications and you want to fully recover, find out why you were prescribed the drugs and work with a qualified health care practitioner to reduce or eliminate your dependency on medications. Every medication, every patented drug, slows or stops metabolic processes. Plus you have to think about this, this is going to sound weird, but back at the turn of the last century, pharmaceutical pills were called *patented medicine*. That means that they had to get a patent on drugs like Lipitor or Prozac. To be patented, a substance has to be completely unique, *something that's never been seen on the planet before*. So this is a completely unique substance, something totally new to the human body that has never been recognized before by a human system. Pharmaceutical drugs are a foreign entity, like an extra-terrestrial – and they're putting it in the human body to alter the physiology of the body. In the future, we're going to think that it's absolutely insane to change human physiology with a chemical that is foreign to the human body and call that procedure "Healthcare." And there's another huge problem: we cannot keep using this type of healthcare that is segmented into different professions: Endocrinologist, Pulmonologist, Cardiologist, Psychiatrist, Gastroenterologist, Dermatologist, Hematologist, Neurologist, etc. That's a fool's approach to healthcare. Each system is dependent on other systems. For an example: if a patient has chronic pain that will cause altered gut function, that can cause altered hormone production, leading to a change in thyroid function, causing adrenal fatigue, etc... To restore health, you have to look at *the entire body*. Shoot first, aim second; or drug first and see how it works out. That is what is happening in health care today too often. The cause or the "why" behind disease is rarely looked for. Doctors today are typically not looking to restore normal physiology and normal function; they are not looking at the whole body or the whole person.

The key to health is using natural products and finding out *what the body is deficient in or what the body is toxic from*. Doctors today need to respect the body and the body's intelligent responses. The new healthcare model will be to look at the whole person and all contributing factors, including the physical, chemical, and emotional stress factors that are contributing to the dis-ease process. At our clinic, we tie it all together. We approach the body with respect and awe, and of course this includes the issue of Depression/Bipolar Disorder. You have to find the body's physical, chemical, and emotional stressors. *This is the key to restore health, and health is the natural state of the human being.*

# Chapter 14

## *Nutrition for Detoxing and Rebuilding Your Body*

As a normal healthy human, you replace one billion cells a day. This massive cell production requires healthy building materials in the form of healthy nutrients. In the U.S.A. today, we have a population that is obese and starving at the same time- starving for healthy nutrients. Anytime you see somebody who is obese, what they're doing is taking in food that they're not digesting; and the body is storing the undigested food. Since the standard American diet is loaded with toxic fats, Genetically Modified Organisms (GMOs), preservatives, and chemical flavorings, this means that the population is toxic. So, we have to deal with these toxicities when we are correcting Depression/Bipolar Disorder.

Your diet needs to be a minimum of 80% plant-based foods and preferably organic. The reason plant-based is important is because there are endotoxins in animal products that can cause systemic inflammation; and this will thicken the blood and increase blood pressure. A plant-based diet also has fibers that clean the arteries.

Eliminate Poly Unsaturated Fatty Acids, also called PUFAs. PUFAs are in almost all packaged foods, and they include canola oil, soy oil, safflower oil, and most seed oils. PUFAs cause blood vessels to clump together. Blood vessels are shaped like a bi-concaved disc, like two Frisbees® glued together. This design holds the maximum amount of oxygen. If the blood vessels are clumped together, they can't hold a suitable amount of oxygen. Note that your brain uses 25% of your total oxygen, so healthy blood is vital for a healthy brain. Also, as the blood gets thicker, your blood pressure has to increase to get that unhealthy blood through your arteries.

For nutrition for normal physiology, you need to get lots of fresh organic fruits and vegetables, eliminate gluten, and eliminate commercial dairy. These are the solutions to healthy self-regulation and self-healing. And eliminate all genetically modified foods, in fact eliminate any processed foods that are not organic.

To regain your health and reverse illnesses like depression / Bipolar Disorder, you first have to look at the nervous system and correct the sympathetic dominant pattern. Correcting the subluxations or nerve pressure is the key to getting the patient out of that fight or flight state. And correcting the sympathetic dominant pattern will restore normal gut nerve supply.

Since it takes about 90 days to heal a gut, for 90 days *eliminate* packaged or canned foods, fast foods, and animal products (meats and commercial dairy).Try to get your food as organic and fresh as possible. The gut is typically very damaged in patients with Depression / Bipolar Disorder, Anxiety, Autism, including many conditions, so you may have to predigest your food to ease off pressure on the digestive system. By predigesting, I mean, juicing and blending. This process breaks down the plants better than chewing and makes it easier to get the healing nutrients out of your food. For healthy nutrition and optimal recovery you need both a blender and a juicer. The best blender is a Blendtec® or a Vitamix®; I have the Blendtec® and I love it. For juicers, I have tried the Champion juicer®, the Breville juicer®, the Green Star juicer®, and the Omega VRT-350 juicer®. My Favorite is the Omega VRT-350 juicer®.

The difference between juicing and blending is that a juicer separates the heavy fibers or insoluble fibers from the small fibers and the soluble fibers. A blender uses the whole plant and most blenders are typically high speed. The advantage of a blender is that you use the whole plant, so it is great for smoothies; and blenders are great for fruits, because with most fruits you want to use the whole fruit to get the best benefits. The disadvantage of blenders is that the high speed tends to oxidize the juice and may destroy some enzymes, and they don't separate the insoluble fibers from the soluble fibers. The process of getting the insoluble fibers separated is vital for *cleaning arteries*. Heavy fibers are great for cleaning *the intestinal track* and very necessary for health. Following is a formula for juicing that I recommend. It is tasty and nutritious juice formula and it produces about ten 32-ounce mason jars of juice:

Three 3 lb. bags of apples

Two 5 lb. bags of carrots

Six bunches of spinach

Three bundles of celery (not three stalks)


If you put the juice in mason jars, and over-fill them so when you put the top on there are no air pockets, and refrigerate them right away, they should stay fresh for between 24 and 72 hours, depending on the juicer. High speed juicers will introduce a lot of oxygen and degrade the juice faster, whereas a slow speed masticating juicer will make the juice stay fresh longer. Get creative on juicing and use a variety of veggies. When you are preparing broccoli, for example, save the stalks for juice. In fact, most of the veggie parts that you would normally throw away are good for your juice. The reason I like the formula above is that apples have malic acid, which is great for cleaning arteries. Leave the core in the apple when you juice. The spinach is loaded with protein; the carrots help with lung function for detoxing; and celery is great for minerals. Add anything else you want: kale, fennel, any dark green veggies.

Blending is great for fruits, and they need to be blended, not juiced. Apples are an exception; you can both blend and juice apples. Blending is awesome for a fast breakfast or a quick meal. One of my favorite blending formulas is:

Coconut Smoothie workout / breakfast:

1 young Thai coconut, 1 frozen banana, 1 scoop veggie raw protein powder, 2 Tbsp raw cacao chips or powder, 1 scoop

spirulina

Here is a useful video on juicing and blending:

http://www.youtube.com/watch?v=INrXthOFQtU

Healthy fats are vital for healthy brain function. Good oils to use are organic cold pressed olive oil, or organic raw coconut oil, or organic palm oil. I recommend on average about 3 Tbsp. per day. Follow your doctor's recommendation for oils; some people may have medical conditions that cause difficulty digesting oils. Coconut oil doesn't require a gall bladder for absorption like most other oils do, so if you have had your gall bladder removed, this may be a good option for you. Coconut oil is a medium chain fatty acid and is excellent for healing brain function. A healthy brain burns glucose, and if there is a leaky gut issue, as there is with most Depression/Bipolar Disorder patients, the large proteins, usually from gluten (from grains) and caseins (from dairy), can attach to opiate receptors (pleasure sensors) in the brain. This action of blocking the receptor sites is very common not only in patients with Depression/Bipolar Disorder, but also in patients with Attention Deficit Disorder (ADD) Autism Spectrum Disorders (ASD). This causes the brain to be almost starved. So it is essential to go on a gluten-free, dairy-free diet and get at least 1 to 5 Tbsp. of raw organic coconut oil a day to heal the brain.

Also, some essential diet changes to help with emotional stressors are:

- Avoid Omega-6 oils (the vegetable oils: corn, safflower, sunflower, canola, soybean and peanut oils), since they greatly enhance inflammation and depress immunity.
- Increase fish oils – sardine, anchovies, mackerel Omega-3 oils micro-filtered to remove heavy metals, or Omega-3's from algae.

Water is one of the most important nutrients! You need to be fully hydrated, which means you need to drink healthy water at the rate of about 50% of your body weight in ounces every day. That means a 200 lb person needs 100 ounces of water every day. Remember, water is a good blood thinner and a great detoxing agent and your body is 70% water. The main problem with the water most people are exposed to is toxins in our water supply. Water today is fluoridated, chlorinated, or packaged in toxic containers. Filtering today's water is vital to your survival and to disease reversal. Water packaged in plastic containers is not regulated by the FDA unless it crosses state lines. I encourage everyone to watch the movie *Tapped* to understand what is happening with the bottled water industry. You need to first filter out the fluoride and you need a filter that eliminates chloride, chlorine, heavy metals, bacteria, and drugs. Healthy water is the key to healthy metabolic function. Below is a talk I gave on the importance of healthy water....

https://www.youtube.com/watch?v=nb6ttXxb5tU

# Chapter 15

## *Sleep Healing*

For recovery from Depression/Bipolar Disorder and to regenerate your brain, it is vital to get deep sleep. The state of deep sleep is called Rapid Eye Movement (R.E.M.). The R.E.M. state is when the body regenerates, and this repair process is essential for healthy brain function. We live on this planet and there are certain rules we have to live with. One rule is gravity; another is circadian rhythms. The latter is a natural cycle that the body goes through and it is vital that you are in deep sleep between 11pm and 1am for optimal healing. No T.V. watching before bed because this puts the brain in a near hypnotic state and can interrupt the R.E.M. state of sleep. If you do watch T.V., then you have to read something (not on a computer but on actual paper) 15 minutes before sleep. Make sure that what you read is not exciting; you want the reading to act like a reset button in your brain so you can get deep sleep. If you have insomnia or take medications for sleep, this will delay healing.

Watch our sleep video for the solution to deep sleep:

http://www.youtube.com/watch?v=FKhdh_GIxKc

Here are some more suggestions for getting deep sleep:

- Listen to White Noise or Relaxation CDs.
- Eat a high-protein snack several hours before bed.
- Don't drink any fluids within 2 hours of going to bed.
- Avoid before-bed snacks, particularly grains and sugars.
- Take a hot bath, shower or sauna before bed.

- No TV right before bed.
- Read something spiritual or religious or uplifting.
- Journaling quiets the mind.
- Sleep in complete darkness or as close as possible.
- Keep the temperature in the bedroom no higher than 70 degrees F.
- Remove the clock from view.
- Don't change your bedtime.
- Lose weight.
- Make certain you are exercising regularly.

# Chapter 16

## *How to Change Your Perception*

The stressors in life can be broken down into three categories: Physical, Chemical and Emotional. We have covered physical stress and chemical stress; now we have to solve emotional stress or your perception. Your perception of your environment is just as important as physical and chemical stress; in fact, it is the *most* important. Your thoughts, or your perception of what is happening, will change how you express health or disease. In science, we know that perception changes physiology; so you can think yourself *well* or you can think yourself into *disease*. Your belief system regarding health, disease and recovery play a vital role in your healing. It takes a huge amount of personal responsibility to take charge of your own recovery. Many people with chronic disease and chronic pain have had their hopes crushed with broken promises of help and recovery that have failed again and again. This is especially true when the disease is labeled as "incurable," which is how Depression/Bipolar Disorder is labeled.

How many doctors have said they could help, only to fail? How many drugs have promised relief, only to decrease some symptoms and cause others? I dealt with devastating injuries and chronic pain for years until I found out that my body could heal. I first had to develop hope; I had to develop a knowing that health was my natural state. When I say "develop," what that means is: you have to work your new thought pattern like you would work a muscle. It might sound insulting to say that disease is partly about a belief system, especially when the daily emotional pain that occurs in Depression/Bipolar Disorder destroys lives and families. Let me be clear: if your belief system regarding any disease including Depression/Bipolar Disorder is that it is incurable, then it will be incurable. Like Henry Ford said: "think you can do a thing, or think you can't do a thing, and you're right." That means your potential for recovery will be dependent on your belief in the human potential for disease reversal. There have been thousands of spontaneous remissions from incurable diseases, and I mean every disease – even cancer. Those remissions first require a change in one's belief system. According to most religions, you are made in the image and likeness of God; and we know from quantum physics that you are more *energy* than *matter*. To breakdown what that means: look at your body first as a collection of organ systems like skin, heart, liver, spleen, etc. These organ systems are broken down into cells; cells can be broken down into molecules; and molecules' can be broken down into atoms; and atoms are broken down into quarks; and quarks are bits of *energy*. So when you view your body, you look solid; but from a different perspective, you are mainly energy. Thought is energy; we know that thought can change physiology. Fear, depression, anger, hopelessness will all cause stress hormones to be produced, and those hormones weaken your immune system response. Joy, hope, love, happiness will all cause totally different hormones to be produced, and these hormones strengthen your immune system response.

Dr. Lorraine Day, with no chemotherapy or radiation, recovered from breast cancer that had metastasized to her chest wall and lungs, and she credits "an attitude of gratitude" as one of the keys to her recovery. I have seen thousands of patients with chronic disease recover, and the one constant is a belief in the possibility of recovery. Even more important is knowing that health is your natural state; all you need to do is correct the physical, chemical, and emotional stressors and then health can be restored. Here are the keys to changing your perception dealing with emotional stress: prayer, meditation, detoxing the body, earthing, and healthy nutrition and supplements. Let's first break down the techniques for dealing with emotional stress, starting with prayer and meditation. Praying daily is the best, and I recommend prayers of gratitude. Since you are a human being, you are made in the image and likeness of God. To acknowledge this relationship is beautiful, and it is essential for an attitude of gratitude. Meditation involves being quiet and concentrating on deep breathing – with an attitude of gratitude for the healing that is occurring in your body. Both prayer and meditation need to be done with the appreciation of the healing already done. There are lots of Biblical references for prayer. One of my favorite stories is when a Roman soldier asked Jesus to heal his servant, and Jesus said he would come to the soldier's house; but the soldier said that wouldn't be necessary, that all Jesus had to do was give the order and the servant would be healed. I like that assuredness that the servant would be healed instantly by just the order of Jesus. Whatever way you choose to honor God, whatever faith you practice, be like the Roman soldier and have the confidence that the healing will occur. Dr. James Oschman wrote the book "Earthing." This is a great book and "earthing" is an excellent technique. The earth has an electronegative charge, and when you have direct skin-on-earth contact, this action has an antioxidant effect on the body. Since chronic pain has an acidic effect on the body – from poor breathing, poor digestion, and altered physiology – changing your system to alkaline will help healing. The standard advice I give to patients is to walk barefoot in the grass or hard sand next to the ocean for 20 minutes. Patients who have diabetes affecting their feet, or some other type of condition that would make walking barefoot dangerous, may be able to just sit in a chair on the grass or on the beach with their feet in contact with the earth. Also, this gets patients outside; the air that is exposed to sunlight carries more oxygen, and direct sunlight (as long as you don't get sunburned) is vital to detox your system and will have a great effect on emotional stress reduction.

Exercise is vital for dealing with emotional stress, but the problem is that if you're in pain, exercise might be impossible. If you are unable to do exercise, just sitting in direct sunlight (without burning) and deep breathing, with your feet in the grass, is a start. As your body recovers, you will be able to do more and more. For example, if you can walk 10 minutes without pain, then start off by walking 10 minutes two times a day. Work up to 30 minutes a day of light walking. As your body heals, you will be able to do more and more, and you will want to push yourself. A good rule is: if you are sore more than an hour after your exercise, you're pushing yourself too much. Here is an excerpt from the British Journal of Sports Medicine:

### *Exercise Better Than Drugs for Depression and*

### *This Will Change Your Brains Structure*

### *Let's Regrow Your Hippocampus!!*

Researchers found that walking for 30 minutes each day quickly improved the patients' symptoms. The results indicate that, in selected patients with major depression, aerobic training can produce a substantial improvement in symptoms in a short time.

In one study that compared exercise with antidepressants among older adults, investigators found that physical activity was the more effective depression fighter.

*British Journal of Sports Medicine April 2001,:35:114-11*

## Chapter 17

### *Colonics, Supplements and Niacin*

With the toxins we have been exposed to, like medications, vaccinations and toxic food, you have to detox. As we age, our digestion changes, so we need to add certain supplements to our diet. Not everyone needs the various supplements we are going to cover; you may just need some basic ones to heal your body and brain. Let's look at vitamin B3, also called niacin. Niacin is one of the nutrients that's depleted when you're drinking alcohol, which is interesting, because alcohol is a depressant, but what do many people do? They drink alcohol when they're sad or depressed, right? Drinking alcohol depletes niacin and depletes minerals. This can cause depression, and if somebody's depressed or anxious, you're also going to see poor digestion and poor elimination.

Poor digestion is going to limit your ability to heal and regenerate. We know that serotonin is produced in the gut, so wouldn't you expect people who are chronically depressed to have poor digestion? Good digestion and good elimination are vital in recovery from Depression/Bipolar Disorder; and niacin deficiencies, along with other B vitamin deficiencies are common in Depression/Bipolar Disorder. B vitamins are absorbed in a part of your intestines called the distal ileum, which is right next to the colon. This is also the most common area for Crohn's disease and ulcerative colitis, so it makes sense that people who suffer from those diseases also have depression and anxiety. This area of your intestines gets its nerve supply from the low back, and if those nerves are compromised or "pinched" that will alter absorption and intestinal function. This is why many people with chronic back pain also suffer from Depression/Bipolar Disorder. Pain is a clue that your body gives you to indicate that there is a problem. However, in today's healthcare system, pain is often treated with medications instead of respected and corrected. If you have a pinched nerve in your back, you may not be able to absorb the nutrients needed for your disease reversal.

One of the most important vitamins for healing is niacin. Depression, headache, confusion, restlessness – these are all possible symptoms of niacin deficiencies. The premier expert on niacin was Dr. Abram Hoffer, a brilliant man and a pioneer in this field. He treated severe mental disorders, including Depression/Bipolar Disorder and schizophrenia, with nutrition, mainly niacin, and of the severe schizophrenics that he treated, 90% recovered. By recovery, I mean they were healthy and free of mental disease. Dr. Hoffer also worked with Dr. Linus Pauling, who won the Nobel Prize twice (which is hard to do). Dr. Pauling also used the term *orthomolecular psychiatry*. Dr. Hoffer and Dr. Pauling respected the fact that the body is designed to be healthy, and if it's not healthy, it's just missing nutrients. It follows that one of the sources of disease, including Depression/Bipolar disorder, is nutrient deficiency.

Other nutrients you may be lacking are digestive enzymes like protease, amylase, and lipase. These digestive enzymes are vital; they are needed to digest proteins, carbohydrates and fats. If you've had a Standard American Diet – the S.A.D. diet – your body is extremely toxic and deficient in both digestive and metabolic enzymes, so you may need to use supplement. Ideally you would get all of your nutrients from healthy food; however, our soil is depleted of minerals, so it is vital that you get a plant-based mineral supplement. I recommend Body Balance® made from sea vegetables and aloe. You can use minerals without vitamins but you can't use vitamins without minerals. Daily plant-based mineral supplements are essential for health. Another good source is healthy salt like Celtic Sea salt or Himalayan salt.

The last part of your digestive track is the colon. The colon is where 90% of your water is absorbed. Ideally you have three healthy bowel movements or eliminations a day. In today's toxic society, regular colonics are necessary for health. So you absolutely have to get the colon clean. I recommend that you prepare your colon with at least three days of a juice feast before a series of three colonics per year minimum. This means vegetable juice. As mentioned previously, there are two types of fibers: soluble fibers that clean out the arteries and insoluble fibers that clean out the colon. Insoluble fibers also help the motility of the colon. Colonics help clean the colon and get the toxins out of your system. Obesity is common in our society today because we are exposed to food products that are calorie rich but nutrition poor. This is the main cause of obesity. Our food supply is neurotoxic and nutrition poor. So most people are toxic and they are starving. That sounds strange that obese people are starving, but if you can't process your food you will store it. Obese people are taking in nutrients and they can't break them down.

# Chapter 18

## *The Summary*

Now you know that emotions are chemicals produced by how your brain is wired. Your brains wiring and structure can be changed; there is a plasticity to your brain and you now know how to change it. You now know that it is not the events that happen to you; it is your perception of those events, and changing your perception is in your control. You now know the toxins that you may have been exposed to and how to detox and eliminate them. You now know how to rebuild your body and your brain and how your nervous system works. Below are the five steps to regain your life and restore your health.

1. Get your nervous system checked for subluxations to get yourself out of the sympathetic pattern.
2. Heal the gut by healthy nutrition, juicing, blending, supplements and eliminating toxic food products.

3. Get your body healthy naturally and work with a qualified health care professional to reduce or eliminate unnecessary medications.

4. Get deep sleep every night.

5. Practice prayer, meditation and exercise to change your perception, and that will change your brain structure.

You truly are made in the image and likeness of God; health is the natural state of the human being. Depression/Bipolar disorder have a cause and that is deficiency and/or toxicity. The solution is in correcting any deficiencies and eliminating toxicities; then the body heals. Don't accept that Depression/Bipolar disorder is incurable. This book has put forward solutions for changing how your brain is wired and the causes of disease. Don't accept a life of pain. You are beautifully and wonderfully made; every person I have ever met is a being of light and energy, and I am truly honored to have laid out some solutions that may make a difference.

Yours in Health,

Dr. John Bergman D.C.

# NOTES